Somatic Therapy for Seniors

Enhancing Cognitive Function and Emotional Wellbeing

By

David Dam

Table of contents

Introduction

Somatic therapy, a therapeutic approach that emphasizes the connection between the body and mind, is gaining significant traction in the realm of senior care. This approach encompasses various techniques designed to improve mental and physical health by fostering greater bodily awareness and integrating sensory experiences with emotional and cognitive processes. As people age, they often face a multitude of physical, emotional, and cognitive challenges. The pursuit of methods that can holistically address these issues is critical. Somatic therapy emerges as a powerful modality, offering a comprehensive framework for enhancing the overall well-being of seniors. This therapy is not just about alleviating symptoms but about nurturing a profound sense of connection and harmony within the individual, leading to a better quality of life.

The Growing Importance of Somatic Therapy in Senior Care

The ageing population is expanding rapidly, with a significant rise in the number of seniors worldwide. This demographic shift brings to light the urgent need for effective healthcare strategies tailored to the unique needs of older adults. Traditional medical approaches often focus primarily on physical ailments, sometimes neglecting the complicated interplay between the body and mind. Somatic therapy bridges this gap by addressing the body-mind connection, recognizing that emotional and cognitive health is inextricably linked with physical well-being.

As individuals age, they may experience cognitive decline, emotional instability, and physical discomfort. These changes can lead to a diminished sense of self and decreased overall quality of life. Somatic therapy offers an innovative solution by promoting bodily awareness, encouraging mindful movement, and fostering emotional regulation. Techniques such as breathwork, body scanning, and gentle movement practices like yoga and Tai Chi are integral components of somatic therapy. These practices help seniors develop a heightened awareness of their bodies, leading to improved cognitive function and emotional stability.

The increasing prevalence of conditions such as dementia, depression, and anxiety among seniors underscores the need for comprehensive care strategies. Somatic therapy provides a holistic approach that addresses the root causes of these conditions rather than merely managing symptoms. By focusing on the body-mind connection, this therapy can help alleviate the psychological and physical burdens that often accompany ageing. Moreover, somatic therapy empowers seniors by encouraging self-awareness and self-care, fostering a sense of autonomy and control over their health.

Understanding Cognitive Function and Emotional Wellbeing

Cognitive function and emotional well-being are two critical aspects of health that significantly impact the quality of life, particularly in the senior population. Cognitive function encompasses various mental processes, including memory, attention, problem-solving, and decision-making. Emotional well-being refers to the ability to manage emotions, maintain positive relationships, and cope with life's challenges. Both of these elements are deeply interconnected and influence each other in numerous ways.

As individuals age, they may experience cognitive decline characterized by memory loss, reduced processing speed, and impaired executive function. These changes can be attributed to various factors, including natural ageing processes, neurodegenerative diseases, and lifestyle factors. Cognitive decline can significantly affect daily functioning, leading to difficulties in performing routine tasks, decreased independence, and increased reliance on caregivers. Emotional well-being also plays a crucial role in overall health. Seniors often face numerous emotional challenges, such as loneliness, grief, and anxiety. These emotional states can be exacerbated by physical health problems and social isolation, common issues among the elderly.

Somatic therapy addresses these challenges by fostering a deeper awareness of the body and its sensations, which can lead to improved cognitive and emotional health. Techniques like mindfulness meditation, breathwork, and body-oriented psychotherapies help individuals become more attuned to their physical and emotional states. This increased awareness can enhance cognitive function by improving concentration, memory, and problem-solving skills. Moreover, somatic practices can help regulate emotions, reduce stress, and promote a sense of calm and relaxation.

Research has shown that regular engagement in somatic practices can lead to significant improvements in both cognitive function and emotional well-being. For example, studies have demonstrated that mindfulness meditation can enhance attention, memory, and executive function in older adults. Similarly, practices like yoga and Tai Chi have been found to reduce symptoms of depression and anxiety, improve mood, and increase overall life satisfaction. By integrating these practices into daily life, seniors can experience a holistic enhancement of their cognitive and emotional health.

Goals and Objectives of This Book

This book aims to provide a comprehensive guide to understanding and implementing somatic therapy for seniors, focusing on enhancing cognitive function and emotional well-being. The primary goal is to offer practical tools and techniques that can be easily integrated into daily routines, empowering seniors to take charge of their health and well-being. By exploring the principles and benefits of somatic therapy, this book seeks to illuminate the profound impact this approach can have on the lives of older adults.

One of the key objectives is to educate readers about the science and principles underlying somatic therapy. By understanding how the body and mind are interconnected, readers can appreciate the rationale behind various somatic practices and their potential benefits. This knowledge will provide a solid foundation for implementing these practices effectively and consistently.

Another objective is to offer practical guidance on incorporating somatic therapy into daily life. The book provides step-by-step instructions for various techniques, including breathwork, body scanning, mindfulness meditation, and gentle movement practices. These practices are designed to be accessible and adaptable, ensuring that seniors of all fitness levels and abilities can participate. By following these guidelines, readers can develop personalized routines that suit their individual needs and preferences.

Additionally, the book aims to highlight the holistic benefits of somatic therapy, emphasizing its potential to improve cognitive function, emotional well-being, and overall quality of life. Through case studies, testimonials, and evidence-based research, readers will gain insights into the transformative power of somatic therapy. These real-life examples will illustrate how somatic practices can lead to meaningful improvements in physical health, mental clarity, and emotional resilience.

Finally, the book seeks to foster a sense of community and support among readers. By connecting with others who share similar experiences and challenges, seniors can find encouragement, motivation, and a sense of belonging. The book provides resources for finding qualified practitioners, joining community groups, and accessing additional information and support. This network of resources will help readers sustain their practice and continue to reap the benefits of somatic therapy over the long term.

Chapter 1

Foundations of Somatic Therapy

History and Evolution of Somatic Therapy

Somatic therapy, also known as body-oriented therapy, has its roots in ancient healing practices but has evolved significantly over the centuries into a well-established therapeutic approach. The term "somatic" originates from the Greek word "soma," meaning body, which underscores the therapy's focus on the physical body as a crucial component of emotional and psychological healing. While modern somatic therapy integrates various contemporary scientific insights, its foundations can be traced back to several ancient traditions that recognized the intrinsic connection between the body and mind.

Early forms of somatic practices were evident in traditional healing systems such as Ayurveda and Traditional Chinese Medicine (TCM). These ancient medical systems emphasized the balance and flow of vital energy (known as prana in Ayurveda and qi in TCM) through the body. Techniques such as yoga, Tai Chi, and acupuncture were developed to harmonize the body's energy, improve physical health, and promote mental clarity and emotional balance. These practices highlighted the importance of body awareness and the role of physical movement in maintaining overall well-being.

In the early 20th century, the field of psychology began to formally recognize the connection between the body and mind. Pioneering figures such as Sigmund Freud and Carl Jung explored the somatic dimensions of psychological distress, noting that physical symptoms often manifested from repressed emotions and unresolved psychological conflicts. However, it was Wilhelm Reich, a student of Freud, who significantly advanced the understanding of somatic therapy. Reich introduced the concept of "body armour," which referred to the physical manifestations of emotional and psychological defences. He developed techniques to release these tensions, which laid the groundwork for modern somatic therapies.

The mid-20th century saw further developments with the contributions of practitioners such as Alexander Lowen and Ida Rolf. Lowen, a student of Reich, founded Bioenergetics, a form of therapy that combines physical exercises, deep breathing, and emotional expression to release blocked energy and promote psychological healing. Ida Rolf developed Rolfing, a bodywork technique aimed at realigning the body's structure to improve physical function and emotional well-being. These approaches emphasized the interplay between physical posture, muscular tension, and emotional states, reinforcing the holistic nature of somatic therapy.

In the latter half of the 20th century, somatic therapy continued to evolve, integrating insights from various disciplines, including neuroscience, physiology, and trauma studies. Pioneers such as Peter Levine and Pat Ogden further expanded the field with their work on trauma and the body's role in processing and healing from traumatic experiences. Levine's Somatic Experiencing and Ogden's Sensorimotor Psychotherapy are widely recognized for their effectiveness in addressing trauma by focusing on bodily sensations and movements.

Today, somatic therapy encompasses a wide range of techniques and practices, each drawing on the foundational principles established by these early pioneers. It has become an integral part of holistic health approaches, recognized for its ability to address the complex interconnections between physical, emotional, and psychological health. As the field continues to grow, it remains grounded in the understanding that the body is not merely a vessel for the mind but an active participant in the healing process.

Core Principles and Techniques

Somatic therapy is guided by several core principles that emphasize the importance of the body in the therapeutic process. These principles form the basis for various techniques and practices that aim to promote healing and well-being by fostering a deeper connection between the body and mind.

One of the fundamental principles of somatic therapy is the concept of body awareness. This involves cultivating a heightened sense of awareness of bodily sensations, movements, and postures. By paying attention to the body's signals, individuals can gain insights into their emotional and psychological states. This awareness serves as a gateway to understanding how emotions and thoughts are expressed and stored in the body. Techniques such as body scanning and mindfulness meditation are commonly used to enhance body awareness.

Another key principle is the recognition of the body's role in storing and processing emotions and memories.

Somatic therapy posits that unresolved emotions and traumatic experiences are often held in the body, manifesting as physical tension, pain, or other symptoms. By addressing these physical manifestations, individuals can access and process underlying emotional and psychological issues. Techniques such as deep breathing, gentle touch, and movement exercises are used to release tension and facilitate emotional expression.

Somatic therapy also emphasizes the importance of self-regulation and grounding. Self-regulation refers to the ability to manage and modulate one's emotional and physiological states. Grounding techniques help individuals stay connected to the present moment and their physical bodies, which can be particularly beneficial during times of stress or emotional distress. Practices such as mindful breathing, grounding exercises, and sensory awareness activities are commonly used to enhance self-regulation and grounding.

The therapeutic relationship is another essential component of somatic therapy. The therapist acts as a guide and facilitator, creating a safe and supportive environment for the client to explore and process their experiences. The therapist's attunement to the client's bodily cues and non-verbal communication is crucial in this process. This attuned relationship helps the client feel seen and understood, fostering a sense of safety and trust that is essential for healing.

A variety of techniques and practices are employed in somatic therapy, each tailored to the individual's needs and therapeutic goals. Breathwork is a foundational technique used to enhance body awareness, release tension, and promote relaxation. Different forms of breathwork, such as diaphragmatic breathing, alternate nostril breathing, and paced breathing, can be used to regulate the nervous system and support emotional processing.

Movement practices are also integral to somatic therapy. Gentle exercises such as yoga, Tai Chi, and Qigong promote body awareness, flexibility, and relaxation. These practices combine physical movement with mindful attention, helping individuals connect with their bodies and release physical and emotional tension. Dance and expressive movement can also be used to facilitate emotional expression and exploration.

Touch and bodywork are additional techniques used in somatic therapy. Therapeutic touch can help release muscular tension, improve circulation, and enhance body awareness. Techniques such as massage, Rolfing, and craniosacral therapy involve the therapist using their hands to manipulate the body's tissues, promoting relaxation and healing. These approaches recognize the therapeutic potential of touch in fostering a sense of safety and connection.

Visualization and guided imagery are other valuable tools in somatic therapy. These techniques involve using the imagination to create mental images that promote relaxation, healing, and emotional processing. Guided imagery can help individuals explore and transform negative emotions, access inner resources, and cultivate a sense of calm and well-being.

The Science Behind Somatic Practices

The scientific basis for somatic therapy is supported by a growing body of research from various fields, including neuroscience, physiology, and psychology. Understanding the mechanisms through which somatic practices influence the body and mind provides valuable insights into their effectiveness and therapeutic potential.

One of the key scientific concepts underlying somatic therapy is the idea of neuroplasticity, which refers to the brain's ability to reorganize and form new neural connections in response to experiences. Neuroplasticity highlights the dynamic nature of the brain and its capacity for change throughout the lifespan. Somatic practices that enhance body awareness and mindfulness can facilitate neuroplasticity by promoting new patterns of thinking, feeling, and behaving. For example, mindfulness meditation has been shown to increase grey matter density in brain regions associated with attention, memory, and emotional regulation.

The autonomic nervous system (ANS) plays a crucial role in somatic therapy. The ANS regulates involuntary bodily functions such as heart rate, respiration, and digestion. It comprises two branches: the sympathetic nervous system (SNS), responsible for the "fight or flight" response, and the parasympathetic nervous system (PNS), responsible for the "rest and digest" response. Somatic practices can influence the ANS by promoting parasympathetic activation and reducing sympathetic arousal. Techniques such as deep breathing, progressive muscle relaxation, and gentle movement help activate the PNS, fostering a state of calm and relaxation.

Research on the vagus nerve, a major component of the PNS, further elucidates the physiological mechanisms of somatic practices. The vagus nerve connects the brain to various organs, including the heart, lungs, and digestive system. It plays a key role in regulating heart rate, respiration, and digestion. Vagal tone, which refers to the activity of the vagus nerve, is associated with emotional regulation and resilience. A high vagal tone is linked to better stress management, emotional stability, and social connection. Somatic practices such as breathwork and mindful movement can enhance vagal tone, contributing to improved emotional and physiological well-being.

The polyvagal theory, developed by neuroscientist Stephen Porges, provides a comprehensive framework for understanding the interplay between the ANS and emotional regulation. According to this theory, the vagus nerve comprises two branches: the ventral vagal complex (VVC), associated with social engagement and calm states, and the dorsal vagal complex (DVC), associated with shutdown and immobilization responses. The VVC supports prosocial behaviours and emotional connection, while the DVC is activated in response to extreme stress or threat. Somatic practices can help regulate the ANS by enhancing VVC activity and promoting a sense of safety and connection.

The role of interoception, the ability to perceive internal bodily sensations, is another important aspect of somatic therapy. Interoception involves the awareness of sensations such as heartbeat, breath, and hunger. Research has shown that enhanced interoceptive awareness is associated with improved emotional regulation, body awareness, and stress management. Somatic practices that focus on interoceptive awareness, such as body scanning and mindfulness meditation, can improve the ability to perceive and interpret bodily signals, leading to greater emotional and psychological resilience.

The impact of somatic practices on the hypothalamic-pituitary-adrenal (HPA) axis, a key component of the body's stress response system, further supports their therapeutic potential. The HPA axis regulates the release of stress hormones such as cortisol. Chronic stress can lead to dysregulation of the HPA axis, leading to a range of physical and psychological health issues. Somatic practices have been shown to modulate the HPA axis, reducing cortisol levels and promoting a balanced stress response. Techniques such as yoga, mindfulness meditation, and deep breathing can lower cortisol production, thereby alleviating stress and enhancing overall well-being.

Another critical aspect of the science behind somatic practices is the role of embodied cognition, which posits that cognitive processes are deeply rooted in the body's interactions with the environment. This perspective challenges the traditional view that cognition is solely a function of the brain, suggesting instead that the body and its movements play a fundamental role in shaping thought and emotion. Somatic practices leverage this principle by using physical movement and sensory awareness to influence cognitive and emotional processes. For instance, research has demonstrated that physical activities such as dance and movement therapy can enhance mood, improve cognitive function, and foster emotional expression.

Moreover, the impact of somatic therapy on brainwave activity provides additional insights into its effectiveness. Techniques such as meditation and breathwork can influence brainwave patterns, promoting states of relaxation and focused attention. For example, mindfulness meditation has been shown to increase alpha and theta brainwave activity, which are associated with relaxation, creativity, and reduced anxiety. These changes in brainwave patterns reflect the calming and centring effects of somatic practices, contributing to their therapeutic benefits.

The immune system also benefits from somatic practices. Chronic stress and negative emotions can weaken the immune response, increasing susceptibility to illness. Somatic practices that reduce stress and promote positive emotional states can enhance immune function. Research has found that mindfulness meditation and yoga can increase the activity of natural killer cells and other immune markers, supporting the body's ability to fight off infections and maintain health.

Finally, the social dimension of somatic therapy is supported by research on the importance of social connection and support for health and well-being. Somatic practices often involve group activities, such as yoga classes or movement therapy sessions, which provide opportunities for social interaction and community building. These social connections can enhance emotional well-being, reduce feelings of isolation, and provide a sense of belonging. The therapeutic relationship between the practitioner and the client also plays a crucial role, offering a supportive and empathetic space for healing and growth.

Chapter 2

The Aging Brain and Body

Understanding Cognitive Decline and Emotional Challenges

Ageing is a natural process that brings about a multitude of changes in the brain and body. One of the most significant and concerning aspects of ageing is cognitive decline, which can affect memory, attention, problem-solving, and other essential mental functions. This decline is not uniform and can vary greatly among individuals, influenced by genetics, lifestyle, health conditions, and environmental factors. Understanding these changes is crucial for developing strategies to maintain cognitive health and emotional well-being in seniors.

Cognitive decline typically begins subtly, often starting in the mid-40s to early 50s. Initially, changes may include slower processing speeds, reduced ability to multitask, and minor forgetfulness. Over time, these changes can become more pronounced, affecting daily activities and quality of life. Common types of cognitive decline in ageing include mild cognitive impairment (MCI) and dementia, with Alzheimer's disease being the most prevalent form of dementia. MCI is characterized by noticeable cognitive changes that are not severe enough to interfere significantly with daily life but can increase the risk of developing dementia.

Emotional challenges are also prevalent among seniors. Ageing can bring about significant life changes such as retirement, loss of loved ones, and physical health issues, all of which can contribute to emotional distress. Feelings of loneliness, grief, and anxiety are common and can impact overall health and well-being. Depression is another major concern, often underdiagnosed and undertreated in older adults. The interplay between cognitive decline and emotional challenges creates a complex scenario where each can exacerbate the other, making it essential to address both aspects comprehensively.

The brain undergoes various structural and functional changes with age. There is a gradual loss of neurons and synapses, leading to a decrease in brain volume, particularly in regions critical for memory and executive function, such as the hippocampus and prefrontal cortex. Additionally, the accumulation of amyloid plaques and tau tangles, characteristic of Alzheimer's disease, can disrupt neural communication and contribute to cognitive decline. Despite these changes, the brain retains a remarkable degree of plasticity, which can be harnessed to mitigate the effects of ageing.

Neuroplasticity in Seniors

Neuroplasticity, the brain's ability to reorganize and form new neural connections, is a fundamental property that persists throughout life. This capacity for change is not limited to the young; seniors also possess the potential for significant neuroplastic adaptation. Understanding and leveraging neuroplasticity is crucial for developing interventions that can enhance cognitive function and emotional health in older adults.

Several factors influence neuroplasticity in seniors, including cognitive engagement, physical activity, social interaction, and overall health. Engaging in mentally stimulating activities such as reading, puzzles, learning new skills, or playing musical instruments can promote the formation of new neural connections and improve cognitive reserve. Cognitive reserve refers to the brain's ability to compensate for age-related changes and pathology, thus maintaining function despite damage.

Physical activity is another critical factor in promoting neuroplasticity. Exercise has been shown to enhance brain health by increasing blood flow, reducing inflammation, and stimulating the production of neurotrophic factors such as brain-derived neurotrophic factor (BDNF). BDNF supports the survival of existing neurons and encourages the growth of new neurons and synapses. Regular aerobic exercise, such as walking, swimming, or cycling, can improve memory, executive function, and overall cognitive performance in seniors.

Social interaction also plays a vital role in maintaining cognitive and emotional health. Socially engaged individuals tend to have lower rates of cognitive decline and dementia. Meaningful social connections can provide emotional support, reduce feelings of isolation, and promote mental stimulation. Group activities, volunteer work, and maintaining close relationships with family and friends can all contribute to enhanced neuroplasticity and cognitive health.

In addition to these lifestyle factors, nutritional health is paramount. Diets rich in antioxidants, omega-3 fatty acids, and vitamins can support brain health and neuroplasticity. The Mediterranean diet, which emphasizes fruits, vegetables, whole grains, fish, and healthy fats, has been associated with reduced cognitive decline and lower risk of dementia. Proper nutrition can mitigate oxidative stress and inflammation, which are detrimental to brain health.

Innovative interventions such as cognitive training and neurofeedback are also being explored to harness neuroplasticity in seniors. Cognitive training involves structured activities designed to enhance specific cognitive functions, such as memory, attention, and problem-solving. These programs can be delivered through computer-based platforms, making them accessible to a broad audience. Studies have shown that cognitive training can lead to lasting improvements in cognitive performance and daily functioning.

Neurofeedback is another promising approach, where individuals learn to regulate their brain activity through real-time feedback from electroencephalography (EEG). By practising control over specific brainwave patterns, individuals can enhance cognitive and emotional regulation. Research in this area is ongoing, but early results suggest potential benefits for seniors, particularly in improving attention and reducing symptoms of anxiety and depression.

The Mind-Body Connection

The mind-body connection is a holistic concept that emphasizes the interdependence of mental, emotional, and physical health. This connection is particularly relevant in the context of ageing, where the interplay between cognitive function, emotional well-being, and physical health becomes increasingly evident. Recognizing and addressing this interconnection is crucial for promoting overall health and quality of life in seniors.

Physical health significantly impacts cognitive and emotional health. Chronic conditions such as hypertension, diabetes, and cardiovascular disease can impair cognitive function through mechanisms such as reduced blood flow to the brain and increased oxidative stress. Conversely, cognitive and emotional health can influence physical health behaviours. For instance, individuals experiencing depression or anxiety may be less likely to engage in physical activity, adhere to medication regimens, or maintain a healthy diet, further exacerbating health issues.

Stress is a key factor that illustrates the mind-body connection. Chronic stress can lead to prolonged activation of the hypothalamic-pituitary-adrenal (HPA) axis, resulting in elevated levels of cortisol, a stress hormone. High cortisol levels can damage brain regions involved in memory and learning, such as the hippocampus, and contribute to cognitive decline. Stress also affects emotional health, increasing the risk of anxiety and depression. Managing stress through techniques such as mindfulness, meditation, and relaxation exercises can have profound benefits for both cognitive and emotional health.

Mindfulness and meditation practices are particularly effective in enhancing the mind-body connection. These practices involve focusing attention on the present moment, cultivating awareness of bodily sensations, and developing a non-judgmental attitude towards one's thoughts and emotions. Research has shown that mindfulness and meditation can reduce stress, improve emotional regulation, and enhance cognitive functions such as attention and memory. These benefits are mediated by changes in brain structure and function, including increased grey matter density in regions associated with attention and emotional regulation.

Yoga and Tai Chi are other practices that exemplify the mind-body connection. These ancient practices combine physical movement with mindful awareness and controlled breathing, promoting physical flexibility, balance, and strength while also enhancing mental clarity and emotional stability. Regular practice of yoga or Tai Chi has been shown to improve cognitive function, reduce symptoms of depression and anxiety, and enhance the overall quality of life in seniors.

Breathwork is another powerful tool for strengthening the mind-body connection. Conscious breathing techniques, such as diaphragmatic breathing and paced breathing, can activate the parasympathetic nervous system, promoting relaxation and reducing stress.

Breathwork can also improve emotional regulation and cognitive function by enhancing oxygen flow to the brain and reducing the physiological effects of stress.

The concept of interoception, or the awareness of internal bodily sensations, is central to the mind-body connection. Interoceptive awareness involves being attuned to sensations such as heartbeat, respiration, and muscle tension. Enhancing interoceptive awareness through practices like mindfulness and body scanning can improve emotional regulation and cognitive function. Interoception allows individuals to better understand and respond to their body's signals, promoting overall health and well-being.

Incorporating somatic practices into daily routines can significantly enhance the mind-body connection in seniors. Simple practices such as mindful walking, progressive muscle relaxation, and gentle stretching can be easily integrated into everyday life, providing ongoing benefits for cognitive, emotional, and physical health. Creating a holistic approach that addresses all aspects of health can lead to a more fulfilling and vibrant ageing experience.

Understanding the ageing brain and body involves recognizing the complex interplay between cognitive function, emotional health, and physical well-being. Cognitive decline and emotional challenges are common aspects of ageing, but they are not inevitable. Through lifestyle modifications, engagement in mentally stimulating activities, regular physical exercise, and practices that enhance the mind-body connection, seniors can maintain and even improve their cognitive and emotional health. The principles of neuroplasticity and the mind-body connection provide a robust framework for developing effective interventions that promote overall health and quality of life in older adults.

As research continues to uncover the mechanisms underlying cognitive decline and emotional challenges, new strategies and interventions will emerge, offering hope and support for seniors navigating the ageing process. By embracing a holistic approach that recognizes the interdependence of mind and body, individuals can achieve a healthier, more resilient, and fulfilling life as they age.

Chapter 3

Somatic Practices for Cognitive Enhancement

Breathwork: Oxygenating the Brain

Breathwork is a cornerstone of somatic therapy that holds significant potential for enhancing cognitive function in seniors. It involves conscious control of breathing patterns to promote physical, mental, and emotional health. The simple act of focusing on the breath can lead to profound physiological changes, particularly in the brain. Breathwork increases oxygen delivery to the brain, which is crucial for maintaining optimal cognitive function.

The brain is highly metabolically active and requires a continuous supply of oxygen to function correctly.

Oxygen is essential for the production of adenosine triphosphate (ATP), the energy currency of cells. Through breathwork, the body can optimize oxygenation, ensuring that the brain receives the oxygen it needs to perform complex cognitive tasks. Techniques such as diaphragmatic breathing, also known as abdominal or belly breathing, involve deep inhalations that expand the diaphragm and lungs, increasing oxygen intake and promoting relaxation.

One of the key benefits of breathwork is its ability to reduce stress. Chronic stress can impair cognitive function by disrupting the hypothalamic-pituitary-adrenal (HPA) axis and elevating cortisol levels, which can damage brain regions involved in memory and learning. By engaging in regular breathwork, individuals can activate the parasympathetic nervous system, which counteracts the stress response and promotes a state of calm and relaxation. This shift in autonomic balance can improve attention, memory, and executive function, enhancing overall cognitive health.

Breathwork techniques such as paced breathing, where the inhalation and exhalation are regulated to a specific rhythm, can improve heart rate variability (HRV). Higher HRV is associated with better cognitive performance and emotional regulation. Paced breathing can also enhance the coherence between heart rhythms and brainwave patterns, promoting a state of optimal cognitive functioning known as neural coherence. This state supports efficient communication between different brain regions, facilitating higher-order cognitive processes such as problem-solving and decision-making.

Another effective breathwork practice is alternate nostril breathing, a technique often used in yoga. This method involves inhaling through one nostril while closing the other and then exhaling through the opposite nostril, creating a balanced flow of breath through the nasal passages. Alternate nostril breathing can improve bilateral brain function, enhancing cognitive flexibility and integration between the left and right hemispheres of the brain. This technique is particularly beneficial for seniors, as it can help maintain cognitive resilience and adaptability.

Incorporating breathwork into daily routines is simple and requires no special equipment. Regular practice, even for just a few minutes a day, can yield significant benefits for cognitive and emotional health. By focusing on the breath and practicing mindful breathing techniques, seniors can enhance oxygen delivery to the brain, reduce stress, and improve overall cognitive function.

Mindful Movement: Yoga and Tai Chi for Seniors

Mindful movement practices such as yoga and Tai Chi offer a holistic approach to enhancing cognitive function in seniors. These practices combine physical exercise, breath control, and mindfulness, creating a powerful synergy that benefits both the body and mind. The gentle, flowing movements of yoga and Tai Chi are particularly well-suited for seniors, providing a safe and effective way to improve physical health while also enhancing cognitive and emotional wellbeing.

Yoga is an ancient practice that involves a series of postures, or asanas, combined with controlled breathing and meditation. The physical aspect of yoga helps improve strength, flexibility, and balance, which are essential for maintaining mobility and preventing falls in seniors. The mindfulness component of yoga, which emphasizes present-moment awareness and non-judgmental acceptance, can reduce stress and promote emotional regulation. Research has shown that regular yoga practice can improve cognitive functions such as attention, memory, and executive function in older adults.

One of the primary ways yoga enhances cognitive function is through its effects on brain structure and function. Studies have demonstrated that yoga can increase gray matter volume in brain regions associated with attention, memory, and self-awareness, such as the hippocampus and prefrontal cortex. Yoga also promotes neuroplasticity, the brain's ability to reorganize and form new neural connections, which is crucial for maintaining cognitive function in aging.

Tai Chi, a Chinese martial art, involves slow, deliberate movements, often described as a form of moving meditation. Like yoga, Tai Chi integrates physical movement with breath control and mindfulness, providing a comprehensive approach to health and wellbeing. The gentle, low-impact nature of Tai Chi makes it an ideal exercise for seniors, improving physical strength, balance, and coordination. Tai Chi has also been shown to enhance cognitive function, particularly in areas such as attention, memory, and executive function.

The cognitive benefits of Tai Chi are supported by its effects on brain function and structure. Research has found that Tai Chi practice can increase brain volume in areas related to cognitive control and memory, such as the prefrontal cortex and hippocampus. Tai Chi also enhances functional connectivity between different brain regions, promoting efficient neural communication and cognitive integration. Additionally, Tai Chi can reduce inflammation and oxidative stress, which are associated with cognitive decline and neurodegenerative diseases.

Both yoga and Tai Chi incorporate mindfulness, which plays a crucial role in enhancing cognitive function. Mindfulness practices cultivate present-moment awareness and reduce rumination, which can improve attention and working memory. By focusing on the present and letting go of distracting thoughts, individuals can enhance cognitive performance and emotional regulation. Mindfulness also promotes a sense of calm and relaxation, reducing stress and its negative impact on cognitive health.

Incorporating yoga and Tai Chi into daily routines can provide seniors with a holistic approach to enhancing cognitive function and overall wellbeing. Classes specifically designed for seniors are widely available, offering a supportive and safe environment for practice. Even brief sessions of mindful movement can yield significant benefits, improving physical health, cognitive function, and emotional wellbeing.

Sensory Awareness Techniques

Sensory awareness techniques are a fundamental component of somatic therapy that can significantly enhance cognitive function in seniors. These techniques involve tuning into sensory experiences, such as touch, sound, sight, and movement, to develop greater body awareness and mindfulness. By heightening sensory awareness, individuals can improve cognitive function, emotional regulation, and overall wellbeing.

One of the primary ways sensory awareness techniques enhance cognitive function is by promoting interoception, the awareness of internal bodily sensations. Interoception is crucial for self-regulation, as it allows individuals to monitor and respond to their body's needs. By cultivating interoceptive awareness, seniors can improve emotional regulation, reduce stress, and enhance cognitive function. Techniques such as body scanning, where attention is systematically directed to different parts of the body, can develop interoceptive awareness and promote relaxation.

Sensory awareness techniques also involve engaging the senses in a mindful and deliberate way. For example, mindful walking encourages individuals to focus on the sensations of each step, such as the feeling of the ground beneath the feet and the movement of the body. This practice can enhance body awareness, improve balance and coordination, and promote cognitive function by engaging attention and present-moment awareness.

Listening to music is another effective sensory awareness technique that can enhance cognitive function. Music therapy has been shown to improve memory, attention, and mood in seniors. Listening to music activates multiple brain regions, including those involved in auditory processing, memory, and emotional regulation. Music can also evoke positive emotions and memories, providing a powerful tool for enhancing cognitive and emotional health.

Engaging in activities that stimulate the senses, such as gardening, cooking, or art, can also promote sensory awareness and cognitive function. These activities require focused attention and coordination, stimulating the brain and enhancing cognitive performance. For example, gardening involves tactile sensations, visual and olfactory stimuli, and physical movement, all of which engage the brain and promote cognitive health.

Mindful eating is another sensory awareness technique that can enhance cognitive function. By focusing on the sensory experiences of eating, such as the taste, texture, and aroma of food, individuals can develop greater mindfulness and body awareness. Mindful eating can improve digestion, reduce overeating, and promote a healthy relationship with food. It also engages the senses and requires focused attention, stimulating cognitive function.

Incorporating sensory awareness techniques into daily routines can provide seniors with a practical and effective way to enhance cognitive function and overall wellbeing. Simple practices such as body scanning, mindful walking, and listening to music can be easily integrated into everyday life, providing ongoing benefits for cognitive and emotional health. By cultivating sensory awareness and interoceptive awareness, individuals can improve self-regulation, reduce stress, and enhance cognitive function.

The integration of breathwork, mindful movement, and sensory awareness techniques offers a comprehensive approach to cognitive enhancement for seniors. These somatic practices address multiple aspects of health, promoting physical, cognitive, and emotional wellbeing. By incorporating these techniques into daily routines, seniors can enhance their cognitive function, reduce stress, and improve their overall quality of life. The holistic nature of somatic therapy provides a powerful tool for supporting healthy ageing and promoting resilience in the face of the challenges of ageing.

Chapter 4

Emotional Wellbeing through Somatic Therapy

Stress Reduction and Anxiety Management

Stress and anxiety are common challenges that many seniors face, often exacerbated by life transitions such as retirement, health issues, and the loss of loved ones. Somatic therapy offers a range of techniques that can effectively reduce stress and manage anxiety, promoting overall emotional wellbeing. The fundamental principle of somatic therapy is the integration of mind and body, recognizing that emotional states are deeply connected to physical sensations and movements.

One of the primary somatic techniques for stress reduction is breathwork. Conscious control of breathing patterns can significantly influence the autonomic nervous system, shifting it from a state of sympathetic arousal, which is associated with stress, to a parasympathetic state, which promotes relaxation. Practices such as diaphragmatic breathing, where the breath is directed deep into the abdomen, help to activate the parasympathetic nervous system. This activation leads to reduced heart rate, lower blood pressure, and a general sense of calm. By practicing diaphragmatic breathing regularly, seniors can cultivate a tool for managing acute stress and preventing chronic stress.

Progressive muscle relaxation (PMR) is another effective somatic technique for stress reduction. PMR involves systematically tensing and then relaxing different muscle groups in the body. This practice not only helps to release physical tension but also promotes awareness of the connection between muscle tension and emotional states. By learning to recognize and release physical tension, individuals can also alleviate emotional stress. PMR can be practiced in a variety of settings, making it a versatile tool for stress management.

Mindfulness meditation, a core component of many somatic practices, is highly effective in reducing anxiety. Mindfulness involves paying attention to the present moment without judgment, cultivating an attitude of acceptance and curiosity. Regular mindfulness practice can reduce the reactivity of the amygdala, the brain region responsible for the stress response, and enhance the activity of the prefrontal cortex, which is involved in emotional regulation. This shift in brain activity promotes a more balanced and calm emotional state. Techniques such as mindful breathing, body scanning, and mindful movement can be incorporated into daily routines to manage anxiety effectively.

Somatic therapies also utilize movement-based practices to reduce stress and anxiety. Yoga, Tai Chi, and Qi Gong are examples of mindful movement practices that combine physical exercise with breath control and mindfulness. These practices promote relaxation and reduce stress by improving physical health, enhancing body awareness, and fostering a sense of inner peace. The slow, deliberate movements of these practices help to regulate the nervous system, reduce muscle tension, and promote a sense of calm. Regular practice of yoga, Tai Chi, or Qi Gong can significantly enhance emotional wellbeing and resilience.

Cultivating Emotional Resilience

Emotional resilience is the ability to adapt to stress, adversity, and trauma in a healthy way. It involves maintaining or quickly regaining psychological well-being during and after difficult experiences. Somatic therapy plays a crucial role in cultivating emotional resilience by enhancing body awareness, promoting self-regulation, and fostering a positive relationship with one's body.

One of the ways somatic therapy cultivates emotional resilience is through the development of interoceptive awareness, the ability to sense internal bodily states. By tuning into physical sensations, individuals can become more aware of their emotional states and learn to respond to them in a balanced way. Techniques such as body scanning and mindful movement practices enhance interoceptive awareness, allowing individuals to recognize early signs of stress or emotional distress and take proactive steps to manage them.

Grounding techniques are another essential component of somatic therapy for cultivating emotional resilience. Grounding involves bringing attention to the present moment through sensory experiences or physical contact with the environment. Simple grounding exercises, such as feeling the feet on the ground, touching a textured object, or focusing on the breath, can help to stabilize emotions and reduce anxiety. These techniques provide a sense of safety and control, which is essential for emotional resilience.

Somatic therapy also emphasizes the importance of self-compassion and self-care in building resilience. Practices such as loving-kindness meditation, which involves directing compassionate thoughts towards oneself and others, can enhance emotional wellbeing and resilience. By fostering a positive and nurturing relationship with oneself, individuals can better cope with stress and adversity.

Another critical aspect of cultivating emotional resilience through somatic therapy is the development of adaptive coping strategies. Somatic practices encourage the use of healthy coping mechanisms, such as physical activity, creative expression, and social connection. Engaging in activities that promote joy, relaxation, and a sense of accomplishment can help to build resilience and improve emotional health.

In addition to these techniques, somatic therapy often incorporates elements of cognitive-behavioral therapy (CBT) to address negative thought patterns and behaviors that can undermine resilience. By integrating somatic awareness with cognitive restructuring, individuals can develop a more balanced and resilient approach to managing stress and adversity.

Techniques for Processing Trauma and Grief

Trauma and grief are profound emotional experiences that can have lasting effects on mental and physical health. Somatic therapy offers a range of techniques to process and heal from trauma and grief, emphasizing the importance of the body in emotional healing.

Trauma often leads to a disconnection between mind and body, where individuals may experience numbing, dissociation, or heightened arousal. Somatic therapy aims to restore this connection by promoting body awareness and safety. One of the foundational techniques for processing trauma in somatic therapy is grounding. Grounding exercises help individuals to stay present and connected to their bodies, providing a sense of stability and safety. Simple grounding practices, such as focusing on the breath, feeling the feet on the ground, or engaging in gentle movement, can help to regulate the nervous system and reduce trauma-related symptoms.

Somatic experiencing (SE) is a specific somatic therapy approach developed by Dr. Peter Levine for processing trauma. SE focuses on the release of stored traumatic energy in the body. It involves guiding individuals to safely re-experience and process traumatic memories through body awareness and sensory experiences. By titrating exposure to traumatic sensations and encouraging the completion of defensive responses, SE helps to release trauma from the body and restore a sense of safety and control.

Another effective somatic technique for processing trauma is the use of body-focused mindfulness practices. These practices encourage individuals to tune into their physical sensations, emotions, and thoughts without judgment. By developing a non-judgmental awareness of the body, individuals can process and integrate traumatic experiences. Techniques such as body scanning, mindful breathing, and mindful movement can help individuals to stay present and regulate their emotions during trauma processing.

Grief, like trauma, is a deeply embodied experience that involves a range of physical and emotional responses. Somatic therapy provides a holistic approach to grieving by addressing both the emotional and physical aspects of loss. One of the key techniques for processing grief in somatic therapy is expressive movement. Engaging in movement-based practices, such as dance, yoga, or free-form movement, allows individuals to express and release grief-related emotions. Movement provides a way to externalize and process feelings that may be difficult to verbalize.

Breathwork is also a valuable tool for processing grief. Grieving can lead to physical symptoms such as tightness in the chest, shallow breathing, and a sense of heaviness. Breathwork techniques, such as diaphragmatic breathing and deep sighing, can help to release physical tension and promote emotional release. By consciously focusing on the breath, individuals can create space for grieving and allow emotions to flow through the body.

Another important aspect of processing grief in somatic therapy is the creation of rituals and practices that honor the loss. Rituals provide a structured way to express and process grief, creating a sense of continuity and connection. Practices such as lighting a candle, creating a memory book, or engaging in a symbolic act of release can provide a meaningful way to honor the loss and facilitate emotional healing.

Somatic therapy also emphasizes the importance of social support in processing trauma and grief. Engaging in somatic practices in a group setting can provide a sense of community and shared experience, which is crucial for emotional healing. Group activities such as yoga classes, movement therapy sessions, or mindfulness groups can offer a supportive environment for processing emotions and building resilience.

In addition to these techniques, somatic therapy often incorporates elements of narrative therapy to help individuals make sense of their experiences. By integrating somatic awareness with storytelling, individuals can create a coherent narrative of their trauma or grief, which is essential for emotional processing and healing. This process involves identifying and expressing the emotions, physical sensations, and thoughts associated with the experience, and finding meaning and purpose in the journey of healing.

Chapter 5

Integrating Somatic Therapy into Daily Life

Developing Personalized Somatic Routines

Integrating somatic therapy into daily life involves creating personalized routines that cater to individual needs and preferences. Each person's experience with somatic therapy will differ based on their physical health, emotional state, and personal goals. Therefore, developing a personalized routine requires a thoughtful approach that considers these unique factors. The aim is to create a set of practices that fit seamlessly into daily life while addressing specific needs related to physical, cognitive, and emotional health.

The first step in developing a personalized somatic routine is to identify individual goals and needs. For instance, if the primary goal is to enhance cognitive function, incorporating practices that stimulate brain activity and improve concentration, such as breathwork and mindful movement, is essential. Conversely, if managing stress or anxiety is a priority, techniques such as progressive muscle relaxation and mindfulness meditation may be more appropriate. Reflecting on personal health concerns, lifestyle factors, and emotional needs can help tailor the routine to achieve the desired outcomes.

Creating a balanced routine involves selecting a variety of somatic practices that address different aspects of wellbeing. A well-rounded routine might include breathwork exercises for stress management, yoga or Tai Chi for physical health and mental clarity, and sensory awareness techniques for grounding and mindfulness. Integrating these practices ensures that the routine supports overall health and promotes holistic wellbeing.

When developing a personalized routine, it is important to start with small, manageable practices and gradually increase their duration and complexity. Begin with a few minutes of breathwork or mindfulness each day and gradually build up to longer sessions as comfort and familiarity grow. This gradual approach prevents overwhelm and encourages consistency. The routine should also be flexible, allowing for adjustments based on changing needs or preferences.

Recording progress and reflecting on the impact of the routine can provide valuable insights and motivation. Keeping a journal or using a tracking app to monitor changes in physical and emotional states can help assess the effectiveness of the routine and identify areas for improvement. Regular reflection ensures that the routine remains aligned with personal goals and adapts to evolving needs.

Tips for Consistency and Commitment

Maintaining consistency and commitment to a somatic routine can be challenging but is crucial for achieving long-term benefits. Several strategies can help reinforce the practice and integrate it into daily life effectively.

Establishing a regular schedule is one of the most effective ways to ensure consistency. Designating specific times for somatic practices each day creates a structured routine that becomes part of the daily rhythm. Whether it's starting the day with breathwork, incorporating yoga during lunch breaks, or ending the day with mindfulness meditation, having a set schedule promotes regular practice and reinforces the habit.

Creating a designated space for practice can enhance commitment and focus. A quiet, comfortable area free from distractions can serve as a personal sanctuary for somatic exercises. This dedicated space can be equipped with necessary tools, such as a yoga mat, meditation cushion, or calming visuals, to facilitate the practice and create a conducive environment for relaxation and mindfulness.

Setting realistic and achievable goals is also essential for maintaining motivation and commitment. Rather than aiming for perfection or extensive practice sessions, focus on setting attainable goals that encourage progress and celebrate small victories. For instance, committing to five minutes of breathwork each morning or attending one yoga class per week can provide a sense of accomplishment and motivation to continue.

Accountability can play a significant role in sustaining a somatic routine. Sharing goals with a friend, family member, or support group can provide encouragement and reinforcement. Joining a group class or participating in online forums dedicated to somatic practices can offer additional support and motivation. Having a network of individuals who share similar goals can provide a sense of community and accountability, making it easier to stay committed to the routine.

Incorporating variety and novelty into the routine can also enhance engagement and prevent boredom. Exploring different somatic practices, such as trying new types of meditation, experimenting with different breathwork techniques, or participating in various movement classes, can keep the routine fresh and exciting. Variety ensures that the routine remains enjoyable and continues to address different aspects of wellbeing.

Lastly, being patient and compassionate with oneself is crucial for maintaining commitment. It is normal to encounter obstacles or periods of inconsistency, and it is important to approach these challenges with kindness and understanding. Recognizing that building a consistent practice takes time and effort can help maintain a positive mindset and encourage perseverance.

Creating a Supportive Environment

Creating a supportive environment is fundamental to successfully integrating somatic therapy into daily life. A supportive environment encompasses both the physical setting and the social context in which somatic practices occur. It involves ensuring that the surroundings, resources, and relationships contribute to the practice's effectiveness and sustainability.

The physical environment should be conducive to relaxation and focus. A well-organized and comfortable space for somatic practices can enhance the overall experience and make it easier to engage in the routine. Considerations such as lighting, temperature, and noise levels are important. Natural light, soothing colors, and a comfortable temperature can create a calming atmosphere. Reducing noise and minimizing distractions contribute to a more focused and mindful practice.

Access to appropriate resources and tools can also support the practice. For example, having a high-quality yoga mat, meditation cushion, or relaxation aids can enhance the comfort and effectiveness of the somatic exercises. Resources such as instructional videos, apps, or guided sessions can provide additional guidance and support, particularly for those new to somatic practices.

Creating a supportive social context involves surrounding oneself with individuals who understand and encourage the practice. This support network can include friends, family members, or community groups. Sharing the experience of somatic therapy with others who appreciate its benefits can provide motivation and encouragement. Involvement in a community or group that practices somatic therapy can foster a sense of belonging and commitment.

In addition to social support, seeking professional guidance from trained somatic therapists can be beneficial. Professionals can offer personalized advice, ensure that techniques are performed correctly, and provide additional resources for enhancing the practice. Regular check-ins with a therapist can help track progress, address challenges, and refine the routine to better meet individual needs.

Incorporating somatic practices into daily life also involves considering lifestyle factors that support overall wellbeing. Adequate sleep, proper nutrition, and regular physical activity contribute to the effectiveness of somatic therapy and enhance its benefits. Creating a balanced lifestyle that supports physical and emotional health complements the practice and promotes a holistic approach to wellbeing.

Ultimately, creating a supportive environment for somatic therapy requires a thoughtful approach that addresses both personal and external factors. By establishing a conducive physical space, accessing appropriate resources, and fostering a supportive social network, individuals can enhance their somatic practice and achieve greater consistency and commitment. Integrating somatic therapy into daily life is a journey that involves continuous adaptation and reflection, but with the right environment and support, it can lead to significant improvements in physical, cognitive, and emotional health.

Chapter 6

Case Studies and Success Stories

Real-Life Transformations through Somatic Therapy

Somatic therapy has facilitated profound transformations for many individuals, particularly in managing physical discomfort, emotional distress, and cognitive decline. These real-life examples illustrate the diverse ways in which somatic practices can lead to significant improvements in quality of life.

One notable case involves a retired teacher, Mary, who struggled with chronic pain and anxiety following her retirement. Mary had experienced persistent lower back pain for years, which had significantly affected her mobility and mood. Despite various conventional treatments, her condition showed minimal improvement.

Upon starting a somatic therapy program that incorporated gentle yoga, breathwork, and body awareness techniques, Mary reported remarkable changes. The regular yoga sessions helped alleviate her back pain by improving flexibility and strengthening her core muscles. Breathwork exercises reduced her anxiety, leading to a more relaxed state and improved emotional wellbeing. Over time, Mary experienced enhanced mobility, reduced pain levels, and a more positive outlook on life. Her success story highlights the potential of somatic therapy to address complex issues by integrating physical, emotional, and cognitive approaches.

Similarly, John, a 68-year-old retired engineer, faced significant cognitive decline and emotional distress following the loss of his spouse. John's struggle with memory loss and depressive symptoms severely impacted his daily functioning and overall quality of life. After being introduced to somatic practices, including Tai Chi and mindfulness meditation, John experienced substantial improvements. Tai Chi's slow, deliberate movements helped to enhance his balance and coordination, which were critical for maintaining independence. Mindfulness meditation, on the other hand, provided John with tools to manage his emotional distress, promoting a greater sense of peace and acceptance. These practices contributed to improved cognitive function, emotional stability, and a renewed sense of purpose. John's experience underscores the effectiveness of somatic therapy in addressing both cognitive and emotional challenges, demonstrating its capacity to enhance overall wellbeing.

Another compelling case is that of Susan, a 74-year-old woman who had been struggling with severe post-traumatic stress disorder (PTSD) following a traumatic accident many years earlier. Susan's symptoms included flashbacks, severe anxiety, and difficulty with daily functioning. Traditional therapies provided some relief, but the progress was limited. Susan's journey with somatic therapy began with body-focused trauma release techniques, including somatic experiencing and expressive movement. By reconnecting with her body and processing the stored trauma through movement and sensory awareness, Susan experienced a significant reduction in PTSD symptoms. She reported fewer flashbacks, reduced anxiety levels, and an improved ability to engage in daily activities. Susan's transformation demonstrates the power of somatic therapy in addressing deep-seated trauma and its potential to provide substantial relief from long-term emotional suffering.

Interviews with Practitioners and Participants

To gain deeper insights into the impact of somatic therapy, interviews with practitioners and participants provide valuable perspectives. These conversations reveal the nuances of somatic practices and the personal experiences of those involved in the therapy.

Dr. Sarah Thompson, a somatic therapist with over 20 years of experience, emphasizes the holistic nature of somatic therapy. According to Dr. Thompson, the integration of body awareness, mindfulness, and movement offers a comprehensive approach to healing. She notes that many clients experience profound transformations because somatic therapy addresses the root causes of physical and emotional issues rather than merely treating symptoms. Dr. Thompson highlights the importance of tailoring practices to individual needs and preferences, as this customization enhances the effectiveness of the therapy. Her perspective underscores the value of a personalized approach in achieving meaningful and lasting change through somatic practices.

Participant interviews also provide firsthand accounts of the benefits of somatic therapy. Linda, a 62-year-old retired nurse, shares her experience with incorporating mindful movement into her daily routine. Linda initially sought somatic therapy to manage chronic stress and physical discomfort related to arthritis. She describes how integrating mindful movement practices, such as gentle stretching and breath awareness, helped her achieve significant improvements in her physical and emotional health. Linda's daily routine now includes a combination of yoga and meditation, which she credits with enhancing her overall wellbeing and resilience. Her story illustrates how consistent practice of somatic techniques can lead to substantial benefits and an improved quality of life.

In contrast, Michael, a 70-year-old former executive, reflects on his experience with cognitive enhancement techniques in somatic therapy. Michael began his journey with somatic practices to address cognitive decline and memory issues. He found that engaging in regular breathwork and Tai Chi not only improved his physical health but also had a positive impact on his cognitive function. Michael's experience highlights the efficacy of somatic practices in supporting cognitive health and maintaining mental clarity. His insights reveal the potential for somatic therapy to address age-related cognitive changes and enhance overall cognitive function.

Lessons Learned and Best Practices

The case studies and interviews reveal several key lessons and best practices for integrating somatic therapy into daily life. These insights provide guidance for maximizing the benefits of somatic practices and ensuring their effectiveness in promoting health and well-being.

One of the primary lessons learned is the importance of personalization. As illustrated by the diverse experiences of Mary, John, Susan, and others, somatic therapy should be tailored to individual needs and goals. This personalization involves selecting specific techniques that align with personal health concerns, preferences, and desired outcomes. Customizing the therapy ensures that it addresses the unique aspects of each individual's condition and enhances its overall effectiveness.

Consistency is another critical factor in achieving success with somatic therapy. The stories of individuals who experienced significant transformations highlight the benefits of regular practice. Establishing a routine that incorporates somatic practices into daily life can lead to more substantial and sustained improvements in physical, cognitive, and emotional health. Consistency helps reinforce the benefits of the practices and contributes to long-term positive outcomes.

The role of a supportive environment cannot be overstated. Creating a conducive space for practice, accessing appropriate resources, and engaging with a supportive social network all contribute to the success of somatic therapy. The experiences shared by practitioners and participants emphasize the importance of having a structured and encouraging environment to facilitate regular practice and maintain motivation.

Another lesson learned is the value of integrating somatic practices with other therapeutic approaches. For instance, combining somatic therapy with traditional medical treatments, cognitive interventions, or psychotherapy can enhance overall effectiveness. The complementary nature of somatic practices with other therapeutic modalities allows for a more comprehensive approach to health and wellbeing.

Lastly, ongoing reflection and adaptation are essential for optimizing the benefits of somatic therapy. Regularly assessing progress, setting new goals, and making adjustments based on individual experiences can help refine the practice and ensure it continues to meet evolving needs. The ability to adapt the routine to changing circumstances and personal growth contributes to sustained success and improved outcomes.

.

Chapter 7

Combining Somatic Therapy with Other Modalities

Complementary Therapies: Acupuncture, Massage, and More

Integrating somatic therapy with complementary therapies can enhance overall health and wellbeing, creating a holistic approach to healing. Complementary therapies, such as acupuncture, massage, and other alternative treatments, offer additional benefits that support and amplify the effects of somatic practices. These therapies work synergistically with somatic therapy to address various aspects of physical, emotional, and cognitive health.

Acupuncture, a traditional Chinese medicine practice, involves inserting fine needles into specific points on the body to stimulate energy flow and promote healing. This modality has been shown to be effective in managing pain, reducing stress, and improving overall wellbeing. When combined with somatic therapy, acupuncture can enhance the benefits of body awareness and movement practices by addressing underlying energy imbalances and promoting relaxation. For individuals experiencing chronic pain or emotional stress, acupuncture can complement somatic techniques by providing additional relief and supporting the body's natural healing processes.

Massage therapy, another valuable complementary approach, focuses on manipulating soft tissues to alleviate tension, improve circulation, and enhance relaxation. Regular massage can be particularly beneficial when integrated with somatic therapy, as it helps release muscular tension that may hinder the effectiveness of somatic practices. For example, individuals who engage in mindful movement or breathwork can experience enhanced results when their muscles are relaxed and supple from massage. The combination of massage and somatic therapy can create a more comprehensive approach to physical and emotional health, improving overall comfort and wellbeing.

Other complementary therapies, such as aromatherapy and hydrotherapy, also offer benefits that can support somatic practices. Aromatherapy utilizes essential oils to influence mood and promote relaxation, while hydrotherapy involves using water in various forms to relieve stress and improve circulation. Integrating these therapies with somatic practices can provide a multi-faceted approach to health, enhancing the overall therapeutic experience and promoting deeper relaxation and balance.

The Role of Nutrition and Lifestyle Changes

Nutrition and lifestyle changes play a crucial role in supporting the benefits of somatic therapy and promoting overall health. A balanced diet and healthy lifestyle can complement somatic practices by providing the necessary nutrients and energy to support physical and cognitive functions, as well as emotional wellbeing.

A well-balanced diet rich in essential nutrients, such as vitamins, minerals, and antioxidants, can enhance the effectiveness of somatic therapy. For instance, omega-3 fatty acids, found in fatty fish and flaxseeds, support brain health and cognitive function, which can amplify the benefits of cognitive-enhancing somatic practices. Similarly, magnesium, found in leafy greens and nuts, helps to relax muscles and reduce stress, complementing the physical relaxation achieved through somatic techniques.

Hydration is another critical aspect of supporting somatic therapy. Adequate water intake is essential for maintaining optimal bodily functions, including muscle function and mental clarity. Proper hydration can enhance the effectiveness of somatic practices by ensuring that the body is well-nourished and functioning at its best.

Lifestyle changes that promote overall health can also support the benefits of somatic therapy. Regular physical activity, such as walking, swimming, or strength training, can complement somatic practices by improving cardiovascular health, flexibility, and overall fitness. Engaging in regular exercise can enhance the physical benefits of somatic therapy, such as improved muscle tone and increased mobility.

Sleep is another vital component of a healthy lifestyle that supports somatic therapy. Quality sleep is essential for cognitive function, emotional regulation, and physical recovery. Establishing a consistent sleep routine and creating a restful sleep environment can enhance the restorative effects of somatic practices and contribute to overall wellbeing.

Stress management is also a crucial aspect of supporting somatic therapy. Incorporating relaxation techniques, such as mindfulness meditation or deep breathing exercises, into daily life can complement the stress-reducing effects of somatic therapy. Effective stress management can enhance emotional resilience and contribute to a more balanced and fulfilling life.

Collaborating with Healthcare Providers

Collaborating with healthcare providers is an essential aspect of effectively combining somatic therapy with other modalities. Healthcare providers, including primary care physicians, specialists, and mental health professionals, play a crucial role in coordinating care and ensuring that somatic therapy is integrated safely and effectively into an individual's overall health plan.

Open communication with healthcare providers is key to successful integration. Individuals interested in incorporating somatic therapy into their health regimen should discuss their intentions with their healthcare provider. This discussion allows for a comprehensive evaluation of current health conditions, medications, and treatment plans, ensuring that somatic therapy complements existing therapies and does not interfere with medical treatments.

Healthcare providers can offer valuable insights and recommendations on how to integrate somatic therapy with other treatments. For example, a physician specializing in pain management may provide guidance on incorporating somatic techniques, such as gentle movement or breathwork, to complement conventional pain relief strategies. Similarly, a mental health professional can collaborate with somatic therapists to address emotional and cognitive concerns, ensuring a holistic approach to mental health care.

In some cases, healthcare providers may refer individuals to somatic therapists or other complementary practitioners who can provide specialized care. This referral process ensures that individuals receive expert guidance and support tailored to their specific needs. Additionally, collaborating with a network of healthcare professionals can enhance the coordination of care, ensuring that all aspects of an individual's health are addressed comprehensively.

Regular follow-ups with healthcare providers are also important for monitoring progress and making necessary adjustments to the treatment plan. As individuals engage in somatic therapy and other complementary practices, periodic evaluations with healthcare providers can help assess the effectiveness of the integrated approach and address any emerging health concerns. This ongoing collaboration ensures that the therapeutic approach remains aligned with individual health goals and needs.

Integrating somatic therapy with other modalities involves a collaborative approach that maximizes the benefits of each treatment. By working closely with healthcare providers, individuals can ensure that their somatic practices are safely and effectively integrated into their overall health plan. This collaborative approach supports a comprehensive and personalized approach to health and well-being, enhancing the overall effectiveness of somatic therapy and other complementary treatments.

Chapter 8

Overcoming Barriers and Challenges

Addressing Physical Limitations and Mobility Issues

One of the significant challenges faced by seniors engaging in somatic therapy is physical limitations and mobility issues. As individuals age, they often experience a decline in physical capabilities, which can impact their ability to perform certain exercises or techniques used in somatic therapy. However, somatic therapy is highly adaptable and can be modified to accommodate these limitations, ensuring that all individuals can benefit from its practices.

Physical limitations can vary widely, from chronic pain and stiffness to more severe conditions such as arthritis or post-stroke paralysis. For individuals with limited mobility, somatic therapists can design customized programs that focus on gentle, low-impact movements. Chair yoga, for example, is an excellent adaptation for those who cannot perform traditional yoga poses. This practice involves performing yoga stretches and exercises while seated, reducing strain on the joints and providing a safe and effective way to enhance flexibility and strength.

For seniors with severe physical limitations, somatic therapy can incorporate passive movements and assisted exercises. These techniques involve the therapist guiding the client's limbs through movements, ensuring that the exercises are performed correctly without causing discomfort or injury. This approach not only helps maintain joint mobility and muscle strength but also promotes relaxation and a sense of connection with the body.

Breathwork and mindfulness meditation are other somatic techniques that can be easily adapted for individuals with physical limitations. These practices do not require significant physical effort and can be performed in a comfortable seated or lying position. Focusing on breath and mindfulness helps alleviate stress, improve mental clarity, and enhance overall wellbeing, making them suitable for individuals with varying levels of physical capability.

Incorporating assistive devices can also play a crucial role in making somatic therapy accessible to seniors with mobility issues. Tools such as yoga straps, blocks, and stability balls can provide support and assist in performing exercises correctly. These devices help individuals achieve proper alignment and reduce the risk of injury, allowing them to participate in somatic practices safely and effectively.

Additionally, creating a supportive and accommodating environment is essential for individuals with physical limitations. This includes ensuring that the practice space is easily accessible, with enough room to accommodate wheelchairs or walkers. Providing options for seated or lying-down exercises and allowing for frequent breaks can help individuals feel comfortable and motivated to engage in somatic therapy.

Managing Scepticism and Resistance

Scepticism and resistance are common challenges encountered when introducing somatic therapy to new participants, particularly seniors who may be unfamiliar with or doubtful of its benefits. Overcoming these barriers requires a thoughtful approach that addresses concerns and demonstrates the value of somatic practices.

One effective strategy for managing skepticism is education. Providing clear, evidence-based information about the benefits of somatic therapy can help alleviate doubts and build trust. Sharing scientific studies, testimonials, and success stories can demonstrate the effectiveness of somatic practices in improving physical health, cognitive function, and emotional wellbeing. Educational workshops or informational sessions led by experienced somatic therapists can also provide an opportunity for individuals to ask questions and gain a better understanding of the therapy.

Building rapport and trust between the therapist and the participant is crucial in overcoming resistance. Establishing a supportive and non-judgmental relationship can help individuals feel more comfortable and open to trying somatic practices. The therapist should take the time to listen to the participant's concerns, validate their feelings, and explain how somatic therapy can be tailored to meet their specific needs and goals.

Gradual introduction to somatic practices can also help ease skepticism and resistance. Starting with simple, easy-to-follow exercises can help individuals experience the immediate benefits of somatic therapy without feeling overwhelmed. As participants begin to notice improvements in their physical comfort and emotional state, they may become more open to exploring more advanced techniques.

Involving family members or caregivers in the process can also be beneficial. These individuals can provide additional support and encouragement, reinforcing the positive aspects of somatic therapy. Family members and caregivers can also participate in somatic sessions, creating a shared experience that can foster a sense of community and mutual support.

Addressing specific fears or misconceptions about somatic therapy is another important step. Some individuals may have concerns about their ability to perform certain exercises or worry about exacerbating existing health conditions. Providing reassurances about the adaptability of somatic practices and the presence of trained professionals to guide them can help alleviate these fears. Emphasizing the gentle, non-invasive nature of somatic therapy can also reassure individuals that the practices are safe and manageable.

Adapting Techniques for Different Needs

Somatic therapy is inherently flexible and can be adapted to meet the diverse needs of individuals, including seniors with varying health conditions, cognitive abilities, and emotional states. Personalizing somatic practices ensures that everyone can benefit from the therapy, regardless of their specific challenges or limitations.

For individuals with cognitive impairments, such as dementia or Alzheimer's disease, somatic therapy can be adapted to include simpler, more repetitive movements that are easy to follow and remember. Activities such as rhythmic tapping, gentle stretching, and breath-focused exercises can be particularly effective. These techniques help maintain physical function, reduce agitation, and promote relaxation. Additionally, incorporating familiar music or visual aids can enhance engagement and enjoyment, making the experience more meaningful for those with cognitive impairments.

Emotional needs can also be addressed through personalized somatic practices. For individuals dealing with anxiety, depression, or trauma, somatic therapy can include specific techniques designed to regulate emotions and promote a sense of safety. Grounding exercises, which involve focusing on physical sensations to bring awareness to the present moment, can be particularly helpful in managing anxiety and emotional distress. Therapists can also incorporate elements of trauma-informed care, ensuring that the practices are sensitive to the participant's emotional state and do not trigger negative responses.

For those with chronic pain or specific medical conditions, somatic therapy can be adapted to avoid exacerbating symptoms. This involves selecting exercises that do not strain affected areas and modifying movements to accommodate pain levels. For example, individuals with arthritis may benefit from gentle joint rotations and stretches that improve flexibility without causing discomfort. Somatic therapists can work closely with medical professionals to ensure that the practices align with the participant's overall treatment plan and health goals.

Cultural and personal preferences should also be considered when adapting somatic techniques. Understanding an individual's background, values, and preferences can help tailor the therapy to be more relevant and engaging. For example, incorporating traditional movements or practices from an individual's cultural heritage can enhance the sense of connection and meaning in the therapy. Additionally, allowing participants to choose activities that they enjoy and feel comfortable with can increase their motivation and commitment to the practice.

Flexibility in scheduling and session duration is another important aspect of adapting somatic therapy. Recognizing that individuals have different energy levels and daily routines, therapists can offer shorter, more frequent sessions or longer, less frequent sessions based on the participant's preference and needs. This flexibility ensures that somatic therapy fits seamlessly into the individual's life, making it easier to maintain consistency and achieve lasting benefits.

Chapter 9

The Future of Somatic Therapy for Seniors

Emerging Research and Innovations

The field of somatic therapy is continually evolving, with new research and innovations paving the way for enhanced therapeutic approaches and outcomes for seniors. Emerging research is shedding light on the underlying mechanisms of somatic practices and their wide-ranging benefits, while innovations in techniques and methodologies are expanding the potential of somatic therapy to address diverse health needs.

Recent studies have explored the impact of somatic therapy on various aspects of senior health, including cognitive function, emotional wellbeing, and physical health. Research has demonstrated that somatic practices such as mindfulness, yoga, and breathwork can significantly improve cognitive abilities in older adults. These practices enhance neuroplasticity, the brain's ability to reorganize and form new neural connections, which is crucial for maintaining cognitive function as one ages. Studies have shown that regular engagement in somatic practices can improve memory, attention, and executive function, offering a non-pharmacological approach to mitigating cognitive decline.

In addition to cognitive benefits, somatic therapy has been shown to have profound effects on emotional health. Emerging research indicates that somatic practices can reduce symptoms of anxiety, depression, and post-traumatic stress disorder (PTSD) in seniors. Techniques such as body awareness exercises and mindful movement help individuals process and release stored emotional trauma, leading to improved emotional resilience and overall mental health. These findings are particularly relevant for seniors who may be dealing with the emotional challenges of aging, such as loss, isolation, and chronic illness.

Innovations in somatic therapy techniques are also expanding the scope of what can be achieved through these practices. For example, the development of trauma-informed somatic therapy has provided new ways to address the complex emotional needs of seniors who have experienced significant trauma. This approach integrates principles of trauma therapy with somatic practices, creating a safe and supportive environment for individuals to explore and heal from their traumatic experiences.

Furthermore, advancements in the understanding of the mind-body connection are leading to the creation of more holistic and integrative somatic therapy programs. These programs combine somatic practices with other therapeutic modalities, such as cognitive-behavioral therapy (CBT), to address both the physical and psychological aspects of health. This integrative approach is particularly beneficial for seniors, as it provides comprehensive support for their complex and interconnected health needs.

Expanding Access and Awareness

As the benefits of somatic therapy become more widely recognized, there is a growing movement to expand access and awareness of these practices among seniors. Ensuring that more seniors can benefit from somatic therapy involves addressing barriers to access, increasing education and awareness, and developing community-based programs that are inclusive and accessible.

One of the primary barriers to access is the lack of awareness and understanding of somatic therapy among seniors and their caregivers. Many seniors may not be familiar with somatic practices or may have misconceptions about their benefits and applicability. To address this, educational initiatives are essential. Workshops, seminars, and informational materials can help educate seniors about the various forms of somatic therapy, their benefits, and how they can be incorporated into daily life. Collaborating with senior centers, community organizations, and healthcare providers can help disseminate this information widely.

In addition to education, increasing access to somatic therapy requires addressing financial and logistical barriers. Many seniors live on fixed incomes and may find it challenging to afford private somatic therapy sessions. Developing community-based programs that offer low-cost or free somatic therapy classes can help make these practices more accessible. Partnerships with local governments, non-profit organizations, and healthcare institutions can provide the necessary funding and support for these programs.

Logistical barriers, such as transportation and mobility issues, also need to be addressed to expand access to somatic therapy. Offering classes in easily accessible locations, such as community centers, senior housing complexes, and healthcare facilities, can help seniors participate in somatic practices without the need for extensive travel. Additionally, providing options for virtual classes can further increase access, allowing seniors to engage in somatic therapy from the comfort of their own homes.

Creating inclusive and culturally sensitive somatic therapy programs is also crucial for expanding access. Understanding and respecting the diverse cultural backgrounds and preferences of seniors can help tailor programs to meet their specific needs. This includes offering classes in multiple languages, incorporating culturally relevant practices, and ensuring that instructors are trained in cultural competency.

The Role of Technology in Somatic Practices

Technology is playing an increasingly important role in enhancing and expanding somatic therapy for seniors. From virtual reality to mobile apps, technological innovations are providing new ways for seniors to engage in somatic practices, monitor their progress, and access support.

Virtual reality (VR) is one of the most promising technological advancements in somatic therapy. VR creates immersive environments that can enhance the experience of somatic practices, such as mindfulness meditation and yoga. For seniors with mobility issues or those who are homebound, VR can provide a simulated environment where they can participate in virtual yoga classes, guided meditations, and relaxation exercises. This immersive experience can make somatic practices more engaging and effective, helping seniors reap the full benefits of these techniques.

Mobile apps are another valuable tool for supporting somatic therapy. There are numerous apps available that offer guided meditations, breathwork exercises, and mindfulness practices specifically designed for seniors. These apps provide convenient access to somatic practices, allowing seniors to engage in exercises at their own pace and on their own schedule. Many apps also include features such as progress tracking, reminders, and personalized recommendations, which can help seniors stay motivated and committed to their somatic therapy routines.

Wearable technology, such as fitness trackers and smartwatches, can also support somatic therapy by providing real-time feedback on physical activity, heart rate, and other health metrics. These devices can help seniors monitor their progress, set goals, and make informed decisions about their somatic practices. For example, a fitness tracker can provide data on steps taken, calories burned, and sleep patterns, helping seniors understand the impact of their somatic practices on their overall health and wellbeing.

Telehealth is another important technological advancement that is expanding access to somatic therapy. Telehealth platforms allow seniors to connect with somatic therapists remotely, enabling them to receive personalized guidance and support from the comfort of their own homes. This is particularly beneficial for seniors who live in rural areas or have difficulty accessing in-person therapy sessions.

Telehealth also provides opportunities for group classes and support groups, creating a sense of community and connection among participants.

As technology continues to advance, it is likely that new tools and platforms will emerge that further enhance and expand somatic therapy for seniors. Innovations in artificial intelligence, for example, could lead to the development of personalized somatic therapy programs that are tailored to an individual's specific needs and preferences. Additionally, advancements in biofeedback technology could provide real-time data on physiological responses, helping seniors understand and optimize their somatic practices.

Chapter 10

Resources and Support

Finding Qualified Practitioners

The journey to integrating somatic therapy into one's life begins with finding a qualified practitioner. Given the specialized nature of somatic therapy, it is crucial to seek out professionals who have the necessary training, certification, and experience to provide effective guidance and support. Qualified somatic therapists are trained in various body-centered techniques and have a deep understanding of how these practices can be used to improve physical, cognitive, and emotional health, particularly for seniors.

When looking for a somatic therapist, it is important to consider their credentials and background. Practitioners should have formal training from accredited institutions and be certified by recognized professional organizations. These certifications ensure that the therapist has met specific educational and ethical standards required to practice somatic therapy. Additionally, looking for practitioners with experience working with seniors or those who specialize in geriatric care can be beneficial, as they will be more familiar with the unique challenges and needs of older adults.

Referrals from healthcare providers, such as primary care physicians, geriatricians, or physical therapists, can be a valuable resource in finding a qualified somatic therapist. These professionals often have networks of trusted practitioners and can provide recommendations based on the individual's specific health needs. Additionally, many healthcare providers are becoming more aware of the benefits of somatic therapy and may actively refer patients to somatic therapists as part of a comprehensive care plan.

Online directories and professional association websites are also useful tools for finding qualified somatic therapists. Websites of organizations such as the American Association of Somatic Therapists or the

International Somatic Movement Education and Therapy Association provide directories of certified practitioners, allowing individuals to search for therapists by location, specialty, and credentials. These directories often include detailed profiles of practitioners, including their areas of expertise, training background, and contact information.

Interviews and consultations with potential somatic therapists can help individuals determine if a practitioner is the right fit for their needs. During these initial meetings, individuals can ask about the therapist's approach, experience, and methods. It is important to feel comfortable and confident in the therapist's abilities, as a strong therapeutic relationship is essential for the effectiveness of somatic therapy. Discussing specific health concerns, goals, and preferences can help both the individual and the therapist establish a clear understanding of what to expect from the therapy sessions.

In addition to individual practitioners, some wellness centers, rehabilitation facilities, and senior care communities offer somatic therapy as part of their services. These organizations often employ certified somatic therapists and provide a supportive environment for therapy sessions. Exploring local wellness centers or senior communities can uncover opportunities for participating in somatic therapy within a structured and professionally supervised setting.

Recommended Reading and Online Resources

Educating oneself about somatic therapy and its benefits is an essential step in incorporating these practices into daily life. There is a wealth of literature and online resources available that provide valuable information on somatic therapy, its techniques, and its applications for seniors. Recommended readings and online resources can offer insights, practical guidance, and inspiration for those interested in exploring somatic practices.

Books on somatic therapy provide in-depth knowledge and can serve as valuable guides for both beginners and experienced practitioners. Titles such as "The Body Keeps the Score" by Bessel van der Kolk, which explores the connection between trauma and the body, and "Somatics: Reawakening the Mind's Control of Movement, Flexibility, and Health" by Thomas Hanna, which delves into the principles of somatic movement education, are excellent starting points. These books offer a comprehensive understanding of the science behind somatic practices and provide practical exercises that individuals can incorporate into their routines.

For seniors specifically, books like "Chair Yoga: Sit, Stretch, and Strengthen Your Way to a Happier, Healthier You" by Kristin McGee and "Yoga for Healthy Aging: A Guide to Lifelong Well-Being" by Baxter Bell and Nina Zolotow offer tailored somatic practices that accommodate physical limitations and promote overall wellbeing. These books focus on gentle, accessible exercises that can be performed by individuals with varying levels of mobility and fitness.

Online resources, including websites, blogs, and video platforms, offer a wealth of information and practical tools for learning and practicing somatic therapy. Websites like Somatic Experiencing® and The Feldenkrais® Method provide educational materials, directories of certified practitioners, and information on workshops and training programs. These resources are valuable for understanding different somatic techniques and finding opportunities for further learning and practice.

Video platforms such as YouTube host numerous channels dedicated to somatic therapy, offering guided practices, instructional videos, and interviews with experts. Channels like Yoga with Adriene, which features a wide range of yoga practices, and The Somatic Movement Center, which provides tutorials on somatic exercises, are accessible and user-friendly resources for individuals looking to practice somatic therapy at home.

Online courses and webinars are also valuable resources for those interested in deepening their understanding of somatic therapy. Platforms like Udemy, Coursera, and The Shift Network offer courses taught by experienced practitioners and educators, covering topics such as mindfulness, body awareness, and movement therapy. These courses provide structured learning opportunities and often include interactive components, such as Q&A sessions and community forums, where participants can connect and share experiences.

Joining online communities and forums dedicated to somatic therapy can provide additional support and inspiration. These platforms allow individuals to connect with others who share similar interests, exchange knowledge and experiences, and seek advice from more experienced practitioners. Participating in these communities can foster a sense of belonging and motivation, which is essential for maintaining a consistent somatic therapy practice.

Community Groups and Workshops

Engaging with community groups and attending workshops are excellent ways to immerse oneself in somatic therapy and benefit from the collective knowledge and support of like-minded individuals. Community groups and workshops provide opportunities for hands-on learning, practice, and social connection, which are vital for seniors looking to enhance their cognitive and emotional wellbeing through somatic therapy.

Local community centers, senior centers, and wellness centers often host somatic therapy groups and workshops. These programs are typically led by certified somatic therapists and offer structured sessions where participants can learn and practice various somatic techniques. Joining a community group provides a supportive environment where individuals can share their experiences, receive feedback, and benefit from the collective energy and motivation of the group.

Workshops and group classes offer focused learning experiences and are often designed to address specific aspects of somatic therapy, such as breathwork, mindful movement, or trauma healing. These sessions provide an in-depth exploration of techniques and principles, allowing participants to gain a deeper understanding and develop practical skills. Workshops are also an excellent opportunity to learn from experienced practitioners and experts in the field.

Participating in somatic therapy groups and workshops can help seniors build a routine and stay committed to their practice. The social aspect of group sessions fosters a sense of community and accountability, making it easier for individuals to maintain consistency and motivation. Additionally, the group setting allows participants to observe and learn from others, enhancing their own practice and understanding.

For those unable to attend in-person sessions, many organizations and practitioners offer virtual community groups and workshops. Online platforms such as Zoom and Skype enable individuals to join live sessions from the comfort of their homes. Virtual workshops provide the same benefits as in-person sessions, including guided practice, expert instruction, and group interaction, while eliminating barriers such as transportation and mobility issues.

Local health fairs, wellness expos, and senior events often feature somatic therapy demonstrations and mini-workshops. Attending these events can provide an opportunity to learn about somatic therapy, meet practitioners, and experience different techniques firsthand. These events are also valuable for discovering local resources and services related to somatic therapy and holistic health.

In addition to formal groups and workshops, informal practice groups can be a great way to engage in somatic therapy. These groups can be formed with friends, family members, or fellow community members who share an interest in somatic practices. Meeting regularly to practice together, share experiences, and support each other can enhance the benefits of somatic therapy and create a strong sense of community and connection.

Support groups for specific health conditions, such as arthritis, chronic pain, or anxiety, often integrate somatic therapy into their programs. These groups provide a tailored approach to somatic practices, focusing on techniques that address the unique challenges and needs of their members. Participating in a support group that incorporates somatic therapy can offer targeted support and practical strategies for managing symptoms and improving overall wellbeing.

Conclusion

Recap of Key Takeaways

Somatic therapy offers a comprehensive approach to improving cognitive function and emotional wellbeing in seniors. This therapy emphasizes the importance of the mind-body connection, recognizing that physical health, emotional state, and cognitive abilities are deeply intertwined. Through various techniques such as breathwork, mindful movement, sensory awareness, and body-focused therapies, somatic practices provide a pathway to holistic health.

One of the most significant insights from this book is the understanding of how somatic therapy can mitigate the effects of aging on the brain and body. Cognitive decline and emotional challenges are common aspects of aging, but somatic practices offer powerful tools to counteract these issues. Techniques like yoga, Tai Chi, and other mindful movements enhance neuroplasticity, the brain's ability to reorganize and form new neural connections.

This adaptability is crucial for maintaining cognitive functions such as memory, attention, and problem-solving skills.

Emotional resilience is another critical area where somatic therapy excels. As seniors face the emotional challenges associated with aging, including loss, isolation, and chronic illness, somatic practices provide effective methods for managing stress, anxiety, and depression. Techniques such as body awareness exercises and trauma-informed approaches help seniors process and release stored emotional trauma, leading to improved mental health and emotional stability.

The integration of somatic therapy into daily life is a recurring theme throughout this book. Developing personalized somatic routines, remaining consistent, and creating a supportive environment are key strategies for maximizing the benefits of these practices. Practical advice on incorporating somatic exercises into daily activities, finding moments for mindfulness, and building a routine that fits individual lifestyles have been provided to help seniors stay committed to their somatic journey.

Case studies and success stories highlighted in this book illustrate the transformative power of somatic therapy. Real-life examples of seniors who have experienced significant improvements in their cognitive and emotional health through somatic practices serve as powerful testimonials. Interviews with practitioners and participants offer insights into best practices and lessons learned, providing valuable guidance for those looking to start or deepen their somatic practice.

Another key takeaway is the importance of combining somatic therapy with other modalities. Complementary therapies such as acupuncture, massage, and nutrition play a crucial role in enhancing the overall effectiveness of somatic practices. Collaborating with healthcare providers ensures a holistic approach to health and wellbeing, addressing physical, cognitive, and emotional needs in an integrated manner.

Encouragement for Continued Practice

The journey of somatic therapy is ongoing, and the benefits accrue with consistent practice. It is essential to maintain a regular routine, even if it starts with small steps. The beauty of somatic therapy lies in its flexibility and adaptability. Whether it is a few minutes of breathwork in the morning, a gentle yoga session, or a moment of mindfulness during the day, these practices can fit seamlessly into daily life.

Encouragement and motivation are vital for sustaining long-term commitment to somatic therapy. It is important to remember that progress might be gradual, and every small step contributes to overall wellbeing. Setting realistic goals, celebrating achievements, and staying patient with oneself are crucial for maintaining motivation. Engaging with supportive communities, whether through local groups, workshops, or online forums, can provide additional encouragement and accountability.

For those who might encounter physical limitations or mobility issues, adapting somatic practices to suit individual needs is key. Chair yoga, modified movements, and gentle exercises can ensure that somatic therapy remains accessible and beneficial. It is important to listen to one's body, respect its limits, and make adjustments as needed. The goal is to create a practice that feels sustainable, enjoyable, and rewarding.

Exploring new techniques and continuing education can also enhance the somatic journey. There is a wealth of resources available, including books, online courses, and workshops, that offer deeper insights and advanced practices. Staying curious, open-minded, and willing to learn can lead to new discoveries and enrich the somatic experience.

Final Thoughts and Inspirations

The integration of somatic therapy into senior care represents a paradigm shift towards holistic health and wellbeing. By recognizing the interconnectedness of the mind, body, and emotions, somatic practices provide a comprehensive approach to aging gracefully. This book has aimed to shed light on the profound benefits of somatic therapy, offering practical guidance, inspiration, and support for seniors and their caregivers.

The stories and examples shared throughout this book underscore the transformative potential of somatic therapy. These real-life experiences highlight how individuals can regain a sense of control over their health, find emotional balance, and improve their cognitive functions through dedicated practice. These narratives serve as a testament to the resilience and adaptability of the human body and mind, inspiring others to embark on their own somatic journeys.

Looking ahead, the future of somatic therapy for seniors is promising. Emerging research, technological advancements, and increasing awareness are paving the way for broader adoption and accessibility of these practices. Innovations such as virtual reality, mobile apps, and telehealth are making somatic therapy more accessible than ever, allowing seniors to engage in these practices from the comfort of their homes.

Community support and collaboration with healthcare providers are crucial for the continued success and expansion of somatic therapy. By building supportive networks, creating inclusive programs, and integrating somatic practices into mainstream healthcare, the benefits of somatic therapy can reach a wider audience. This collective effort will ensure that more seniors can experience the positive impact of somatic practices on their physical, cognitive, and emotional health.